Title: Slimming Strategies: Embrace Small Daily Changes for Weight Loss Success

George E. Morris

INTRODUCTION..**4**

CHAPTER 1.. **8**

CHAPTER 2..**11**

CHAPTER 3... **16**

CHAPTER 4.. **23**

CHAPTER 5.. **27**

CHAPITRE 6... **32**

CHAPTER 7... **45**

CHAPTER 8... **52**

CHAPTER 9... **60**

Creating a Support System......................................60

CHAPTER 10... **64**

INTRODUCTION

Why you need slimming strategies

Use these tried- and-true styles to lose weight and ameliorate your health.

There are hundreds of style diets, weight-reduction schemes, and blatant swindles that promise quick and royal weight loss. Still, a balanced, calorie- controlled diet combined with increased physical exertion remains the foundation of successful weight loss. Endless adaptations in your life and health actions are needed for long- term weight loss success. How do you make long- term changes? Consider using these weight- loss tactics to achieve success

1. Make certain that you're set. Long- term weight loss requires time, work, and fidelity. While you do not want to put off losing weight indefinitely, you should be sure you are ready to make long- term adaptations to your diet and physical exertion habits. To determine your readiness, ask yourself the following questions: Is it possible for me to reduce weight? Are other pressures causing me to become distracted? Do I use food to help me manage with stress?Is it time for me to learn or employ new stress- **operation techniques?**Do I need fresh help, either from musketeers or professionals, to deal with stress? Am I willing to alter my eating habits? Is it possible for me to change my exertion habits? Do I've the time to devote to making these variations? Consult your croaker if you need backing running pressures or feelings that appear to be impediments to your medication. When you are ready, setting pretensions, staying married, and changing habits will be easy.

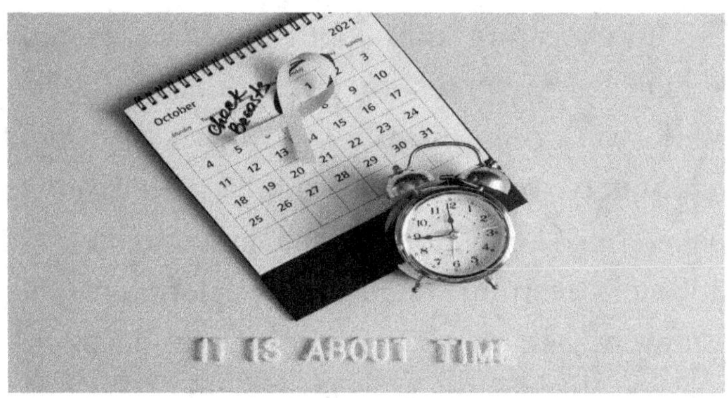

No order to lose weight successfully, having the applicable kind of support can help. Choose people who'll encourage you in a positive way, without shame, embarrassment, or sabotage. Find people who'll listen to your enterprises and studies, spend time exercising with you or making nutritional fashions, and partake in your commitment to living a healthier life. Your support group can also give responsibility, which can be an important motivator for staying on track with your weight- loss pretensions. Still, hold yourself responsible by having frequent weigh- sways, keeping a journal of your diet and exercise sweats, If you choose to keep your weight- loss intentions private.

CHAPTER 1

Understanding the Weight Loss Journey,

It's tempting to compare oneself to others, especially in the age of social media. Your trip is all yours. rather than being forced to feel shy because of what you see others negotiating, concentrate on where you're and ameliorate from there. This applies to all angles of good, whether you are trying out a new strength training authority or changing your food habits. Just because you can not perform a tough action, similar to a dumbbell catch, does not indicate you will not get there one day. Consume proteins, fats, and vegetables. At each mess, try to include a variety of foods. Make trouble moving your body. For maximum health, the Physical exertion Guidelines for Americans endorse mixing cardio exercises with weight training.

 • Consume further fiber.
 • Eat sluggishly and designedly.
 • Keep doused .
 • Get enough sleep.

Losing weight is primarily an interior problem. You'll lose hard fat that surrounds your organs similar to the liver and feathers first, followed by soft fat similar to midriff and ham fat. Fat loss around the organs causes you to come slender and stronger. Set a time limit for your ideal to measure your progress.(For illustration, by the end of May, I plan to walk to work twice a week.) Flash back that the most effective approach to lose weight is to do so gradually by making small, manageable changes to your diet and physical exertion routines. Set yourself one or two minor changes to work on at a time, adding to these only formerly they've come your new way of life. Be gentle with yourself; if effects do not go as planned, keep trying. You may need to revise your pretensions or the time needed to reach them.

CHAPTER 2

SETTING GOALS

The first step in a new weight reduction hunt is determining how important weight you want to reduce. There are multitudinous approaches to developing a long- term end that's both realistic and aspirational. Setting pretensions for the future can help you find the drive you need to make healthy choices. Then is where to begin. numerous people believe they should reduce weight, indeed if this isn't always the case. It's common to have an exaggerated idea of what constitutes a healthy weight. There are several factors to consider while deciding whether or not to lose weight for health reasons. A suitable seeker for weight loss may have the following measures in general BMI lesser than or equal to 25 Circumference of the midriff further than 35-inch abdominal circumference in women and 40-inch abdominal circumference in malesWaist-to- hipsterism rate lesser than 0.8 for women and lesser than 1.0 for malesBody Mass Index(BMI) is an outmoded, slanted standard that ignores colorful aspects similar as body composition, race, race, gender, bandage.Despite being a defective measure, BMI is constantly employed in the medical field moment since it's a cheap and rapid-fire way to assess possible health status and outcomes.However, a modest thing of 5 to 10 of your current weight can start to ameliorate crucial signs like blood pressure and blood sugar situations, If you are trying to lose weight for health reasons.3 Other advantages of indeed mild weight loss include increased energy, further tone- confidence, lesser fitness, and enhanced mobility. Still, our pretensions are occasionally motivated by other considerations, similar to the desire to fit back into old clothes or to appear a specific way. There is nothing wrong with setting a vanity thing as long as it's realistic and does not lead to dangerous light. You and your health care provider can decide whether it's a suitable time to set a weight loss goal.

Setting SMART Goals

The key to setting weight reduction pretensions is to cleave to the thing- **setting** criteria, which means they must be **SMART. A SMART** thing is defined as having the following characteristics: Make your end apparent by using statistics and details in your thing.

Measurable: How will you cover your progress? Will you take body weight, midriff circumference, or exercise performance measures?

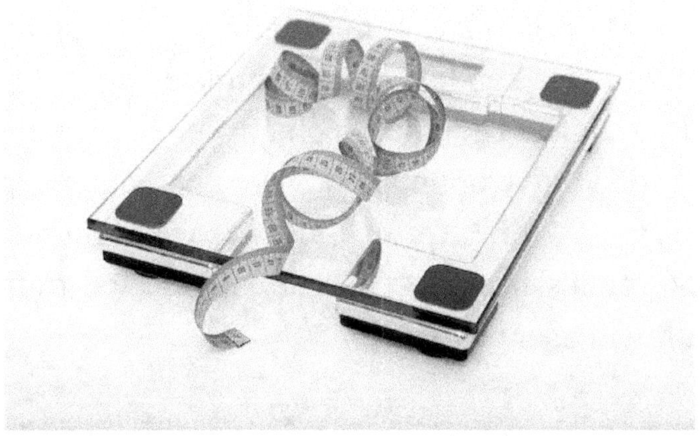

Attainable Do you have the necessary time, coffers, and provocation to complete your task?

Realistic. It's fine to establish a lofty end as long as it's doable and attainable.

Time- bound Give your thing a deadline. To keep on track for the long haul, divide it into shorter- term mileposts. The most important thing to flash back is that lasting weight loss takes time. •

Establishing Your Ideal Body Another important aspect of nutrition assessment is estimating normal and optimal body weight. This enables the computation of the chance weight shift from real to typical body weight. The weight- height reference map produced from Metropolitan Life Insurance Company actuarial data can be used to estimate applicable body weight. The Metropolitan height- weight maps don't give optimal body weights for people of color or from low socioeconomic backgrounds because the data is collected from healthy men and women.

CHAPTER 3

Changing Your Attitude

Losing weight begins in your mind. Yes, you read that correctly! While diet and exercise are important components of any weight loss journey, the actual magic occurs in your head. Many mentality modifications must be considered in order to achieve long-term success. Are you interested in learning how to prepare your mind for weight loss? Let's speak about mindset if you're ready to kickstart your weight reduction journey!

Why is mentality important

Down from nutrition and exercise, there is another factor that is critical to weight loss success. This is your frame of thinking. When trying to lose weight, it's critical that you are in the applicable frame of mind. Mindset is important since it will get you through delicate times. What exactly do I mean? Consider occasions in the history when you sought to lose weight. What were your studies? Were you put off by a slow scale? What kind of tone- talk did you engage in? While this may appear insignificant, I assure you that it's not. How we communicate to ourselves has a direct impact on our conduct, which produce our results. Take a look at the graph to observe how your studies will affect your issues. What do you suppose would be if you woke up one morning, hopped on the scale, and saw a larger number than you anticipated? With the traditional" chooser's mindset," you can feel frustrated and suppose," I'll norway get to my thing." This thinking creates a sense of failure. It's not easy to feel like a failure. As you go about your day, this mood may impact your conduct and beget you to give up, believing that eating healthy is" pointless" because the scale isn't moving anyway. In this situation, the prospect of norway completing your ideal created a sense of failure, which impacted your conduct to abandon healthy eating. But what if you had another idea? What if, after seeing that lower number, you realized that weight loss is not a direct process? perhaps your study would be," This is just a temporary moment and will not determine my long- term success." Every day, I work toward my objects." That first allowed might have made you feel more encouraged, right? People who are encouraged make better opinions. The study of working towards your thing made you feel encouraged, herding you to act in a way that will help you achieve your points. Do you see how your studies have an effect on your results? If you're looking for ways to put this generality into action, I've got you covered! moment, we're diving deep into the station and examining eight critical differences for anyone trying to lose weight. redirect your attention When trying to reduce weight, it's easy to get caught up in the physical element of it. rather, strive to enhance your nutrition and life in order to alleviate your general health or illness troubles. It makes natural provocation less obvious. There are several excellent styles for doing so, but my particular favorite is to begin by journaling. Consider some of the other driving aspects in your life for being healthy. This could be to improve your health parameters, have farther energy to play with your children, have lower tone- confidence, or just to stretch life. Whatever it is, consider some of the goods that are important to you and spend some time journaling about why these goods are significant to you. When you're feeling unmotivated to stick to your health plan, relate back to this list and suppose on why you should keep going.

Select sustainability over speed.

So Numerous style diets and trends encourage quick weight loss. These rules, still, are bad for your overall health because they vitiate your energy situations and performance. It's further vital to borrow long- term actions that will help you lose weight rather than a fast, dangerous fix. While it may be tempting to try the rearmost crash diet in order to squeeze into a dress for a particular occasion, keep in mind that these diets don't promote long- term heartiness. numerous of these" quick results" plans will leave you more frustrated and depleted than when you began. rather than following the rearmost trend, consider making long- term health adaptations. Consider whether it's a commodity you can picture yourself doing in the long run.However, it's time to make a change, If not.

The key to success is consistency.

As we bandied over in the illustration, weight loss isn't a direct process. You'll have lapses and glitches, but what matters is that you keep showing up. When these potholes appear, keep in mind that you are still on the right track. Every day, take one small step closer to your ideal by taking patient action. You could consider adding the following little stages to your routine Every week, I try one new veggie. Drinking acceptable water for your body on a diurnal base Walking for 10 twinkles in the morning and evening These sweats may appear insignificant, but steady, bitsy ways are significantly more salutary than erratic dashes toward your thing.

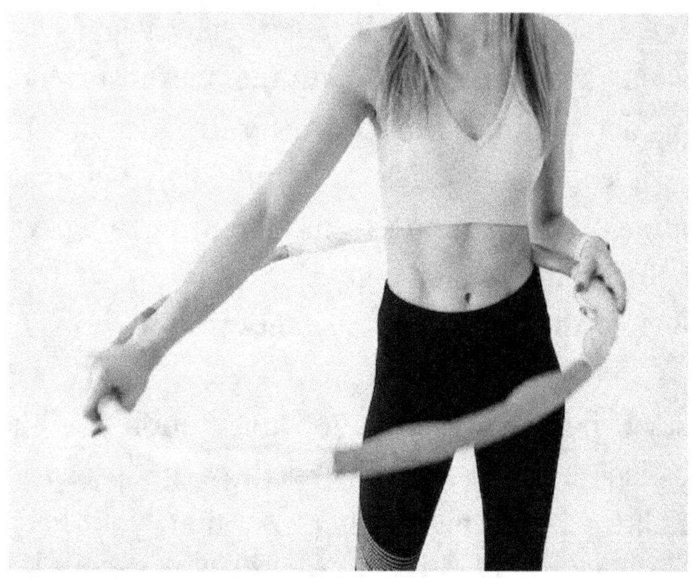

CHAPTER 4

Creating a Healthy Diet Plan

Planning ahead of time will help you eat nutritional reflections and snacks no matter how excited your schedule becomes. A mess plan can help you save time, plutocrat, and help food waste. Just keep your shopping list in mind The following are the six way to creating a food plan

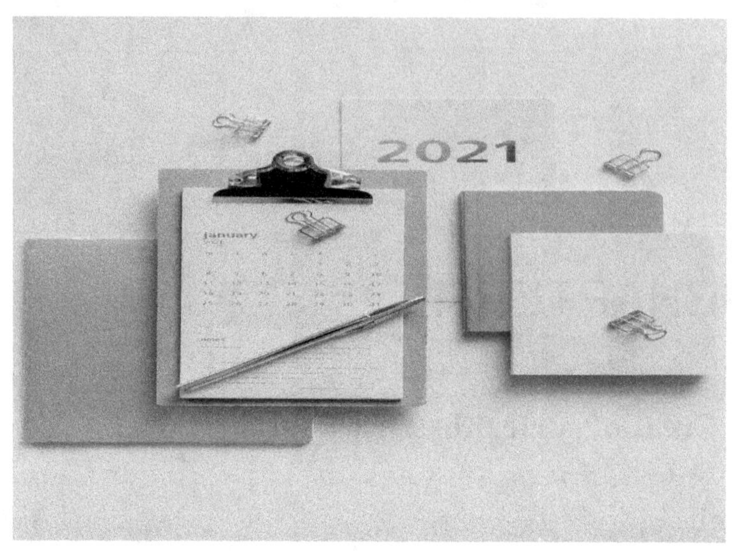

1. Allow yourself enough time to plan.

Make a mess plan at least once a week. Consider the following: How many reflections do you need to cook for the week? When you need to prepare reflections snappily or in advance

2. twice- check your inventories.

Examine what constituents you formerly have in your closet, refrigerator, or freezer. Check the list of foods to see what needs to be used up first, and also arrange your reflections around that. The manner you store food has a significant impact on how long it'll survive. Follow these guidelines Check the marker for storehouse instructions. Place new goods in the reverse of the fridge/ cupboard and aged particulars in the front. Before freezing, mark all foods with their names and dates so they may be fluently linked.

3. Include some of your favorite dishes.

Make a list of your favorite foods. When you have fresh time, try out different fashions. Consider having a themed night, similar to Meatless Monday.

4. Make use of any leaving Plan.

reflections that can be cooled and reheated or eaten cold the following day, similar as pasta singe, haze, cowgirl's pie, curry, lasagne, or beef stew. Make an omelet, haze, or salad with leftover vegetables, or add leftover meat to a curry or stir- shindig. Flash back that leaves in the fridge must be consumed within three days.

5. Make a lot of food.

Cook redundant and store the leaves in the refrigerator or freezer. Pies, curries, stews, and salvers each keep nicely in the freezer. Consider what differently you can cook at the same time if you are using the oven.However, cook some funk guts for sandwiches, If you are making a dish.

6. Make your constituents work together fashions.

that use the same essential constituents, similar as repast funk, funk stir shindig, and funk sandwiches, should be chosen. Choose 2- 3 primary veggies and combine them with a meat, pasta, or seafood mess. Peppers, broccoli, and sweetcorn, for illustration, can be added to a beef stir- shindig but also used to make a vegetable pasta singe or eaten with meat or fish.

CHAPTER 5

Creating Effective Exercise Routines

Creating a fitness training plan that's targeted to your specific pretensions will increase your chances of success. The key to creating an effective training plan is to identify your pretensions, elect the applicable conditioning, and track your progress along the way. You will be well on your way to reaching your fitness objects if you negotiate these effects and stick to your plan.

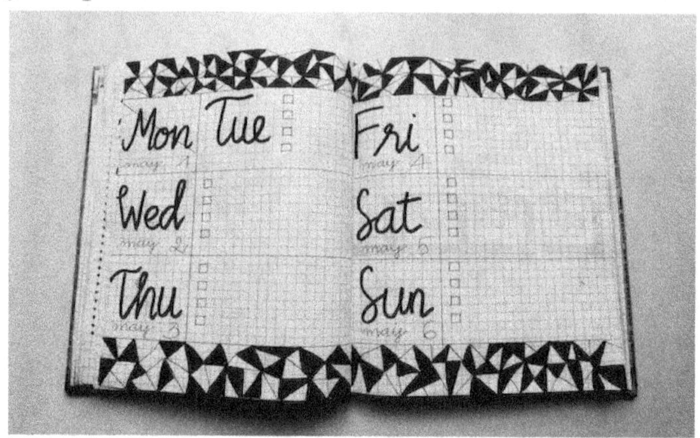

1. Setting Your Pretensions produce.

a list of your particular fitness objectives.Putting your pretensions on paper will make it easier to produce a training plan around them. Take the time to consider what you want to negotiate with your training strategy. For example, you could want to reduce 20 pounds(9.1 kg) or acquire 25 pounds(11 kg) of muscular mass. Your end could be as simple as feeling further energized and attentive during the day, or as complex as boosting your mood through exercise.

2. Develop a realistic schedule for attaining your objects.

The timeline for your fitness training plan is determined by your unique pretensions. Setting a schedule will help you record your exercises and stay on track. Set short- term and medium- term pretensions to help you stay motivated as you work toward your long- term pretensions. For illustration, you may set a goal of running a 1K race or running three days out of seven. For example, if you want to lose 10 pounds(4.5 kg), your time frame could be two months. Because you can lose 1- 2 pounds(0.45-0.91 kg) per week at a healthy rate, two months is a reasonable time frame. Still, you may set a reasonable target of adding 1- 2 pounds(0, If you want to make muscle mass.45-0.91 kg) of muscle mass every month. Still, similar to adding your allowance so you can go touring further, try to resolve them up into lower supplements, If you have long- term fitness objectives. For illustration, after three months, you might want to go on a one- afar(1.6- kilometer) hike, and after six months, you might want to go on a three- afar(4.8-kilometer) hike.

3. Determine your current position of fitness.

Before you start designing your fitness training plan, you should determine your current position of physical fitness. Also you can compare your data along the way to your morning point to see how far you've progressed. Weigh yourself and put down your starting weight if you want to lose or gain weight. You might also use a measuring tape recording to take body measures to see how your body changes. Before you begin training, note how important weight you can lift if you are erecting a fitness plan to get stronger and make muscular mass. Before you begin, take a picture of yourself. Take another print every 2-4 weeks to track your enhancement. still, walk or run afar and time yourself, If you want to enhance your abidance. You can also measure and keep track of your BMI.

4. Make nutritional changes to help you reach your fitness goals.

While regular exercise might help you achieve your goals, you should also consider eating a better diet, especially if you are trying to exfoliate weight or gain muscle mass. Eating healthier foods will offer you further energy for your exercises and allow you to see benefits briskly. Still, limit your input of sticky and salty reused foods, If you are trying to reduce weight. Replace reused foods with fruits and vegetables, as well as foods high in healthy fats, similar to olive oil painting, avocados, salmon, and nuts. Fat protein-rich foods like funk, eggs, rubbish, and sap if you want to increase muscle mass. Every day, end for0.6- 1 gram of protein for 1 pound(0.45 kg) of body weight.

CHAPITRE 6

OVERCOMING DIFFICULTIES

But, when it comes to losing weight, we want results, do not we? Then are the most common weight- loss roadblocks and how to overcome them.

1. you're unfit to stop munching in between reflections.

I understand; utmost of us are savorers who can not go long ages without eating. This was also one of my main walls to losing weight. I'm someone who needs alignment on a regular basis. Indeed if you serve me a large lunch, I'll most clearly ask for a commodity within the coming two hours. So, rather of eating whatever comes to hand and feeling terrible latterly, I could organize my snacks like I do my breakfast, lunch, and supper. At work, it's chips from a dealing machine; at home, it's ice cream from the freezer or other closet delicacies. In my opinion, pure white rice is sufficient. These were and continue to be my roadblocks. result Examine your eating habits and favorite foods. Make a list of low- calorie healthy snacks ahead of time. Include snacks in your diurnal diet, just as you should know that you have a time niche for snacks like you do for lunch and regale. This will help you control your urges and unplanned eating. When you know food is staying for you, you're less likely to eat anything that isn't necessary for your body. Apples, handwrought chips, indeed a bitsy volume of manual fried rice, watermelon sticks, single toast with peanut adulation, manual nut bars, savory balls, and falafel are all respectable. Actually, there's no detriment in eating at the store- bought chips like multigrain crisps or potato chips. If only you could plan ahead of time and stick to it. When you do not plan ahead of time, you end up eating further than you need.

2 after supper or late at night snacking.

result I would recommend repeating the below exertion. Plan your day so that you can have a snack after regale. Your mind will be pleased because it's now wired to anticipate a pleasure after regale. Still, drink warm milk or a healthy treat like chia seed pudding or low- calorie chocolate scum, If you are working late. Another option is to stick to a schedule and go to bed at a reasonable hour. The utmost food accidents after supper(at least in my experience) occur when you continually use social media and get tired of not having any new updates to watch and calculate on food.

3. you're unfit to stop consuming alcohol.

This inordinate drinking habit is one of several challenges to losing weight.And numerous people fail to overcome this because they try to DEPRIVE themselves entirely. There's no need to completely hesitate from alcohol or carbonated drinks. Begin by limiting your daily alcohol consumption. Talk it over with your musketeers and hold yourself responsible to them. Rather, why not try mocktails and manual cold drinks with a hint of alcohol? Inform your musketeers that you're trying to reduce weight so that they won't force you to drink at gatherings. When going out, be prepared to say no and exploration druthers

ahead of time. Eat a healthy diet and go to bed beforehand to avoid the necessity and temptation of late- night alcohol consumption.

4.You   don't   have   time   to   cook

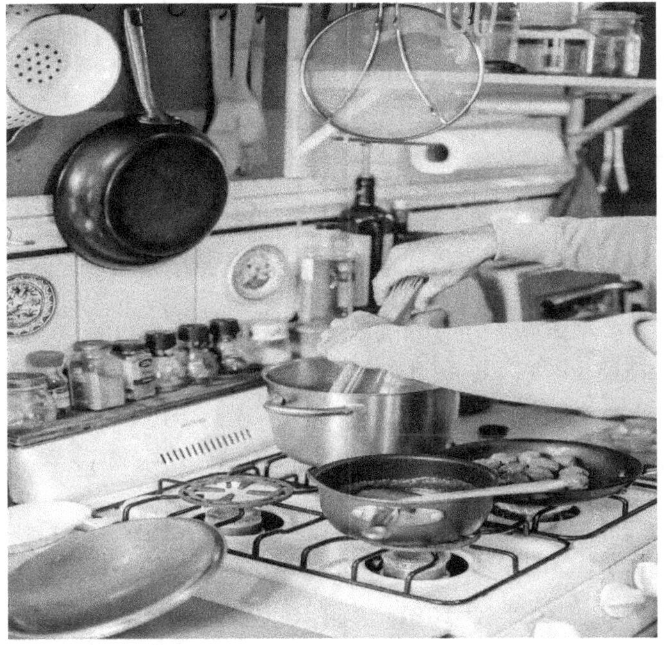

PREPARE, is your ultimate answer. Meal prep is your buddy; there is no reason not to devote a day or two every week to preparing your food for the entire week. Preparing all of my meals or at least the components for the entire week has been really beneficial to my weight reduction journey.Cook and store grains like rice, quinoa, potatoes, and couscous in airtight containers.Make curries, dals, sautéed vegetables, boiled eggs, poultry, and other dishes to go with your favorite grains. I also boil pulses such as chickpeas and beans to use in stews, salads, and curries throughout the week. You do not need to prepare a full meal ahead of time; simply cut your vegetables, boil pulses, grill chicken, and prepare a meal when you are ready to eat.

Here's a screenshot of my supper prep from my Instagram page for you. If you don't already follow me, please do so so that you can get similar meal prep ideas and many more.

I also attempted to prepare my smoothie bags ahead of time so that I could leave them out for an hour while I prepared. Then I'll make my smoothie and go to work. It's that simple if you've mastered meal preparation

5.you cannot afford to join a gym

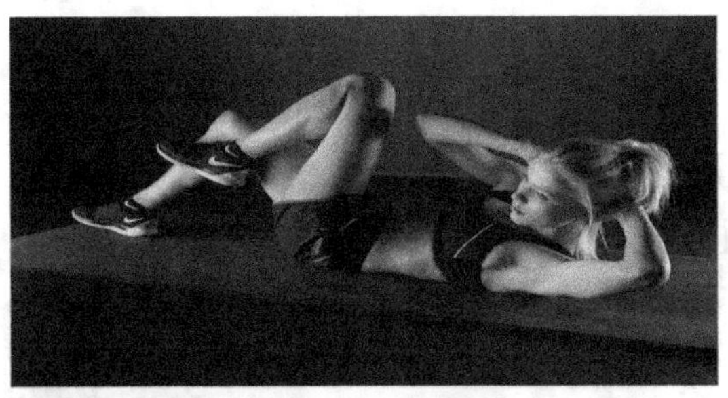

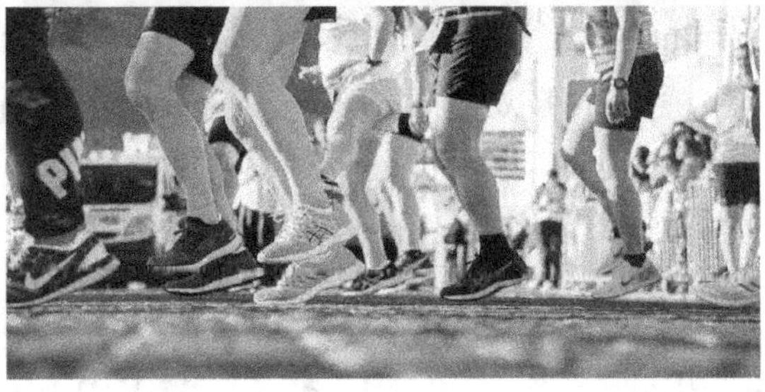

One of the most prevalent barriers to weight loss is a lack of physical activity. But it isn't because I go to the gym. You can lose weight without going to the gym.Walking, running, and cycling are the most inexpensive and free ways to receive enough physical exercise while also breathing in fresh air in nature.

There are various free workouts on YouTube, such as this Fitness Blender, which provides a step-by-step guidance to getting started with exercise to lose weight. Choose one that is convenient for you and your schedule, stick to it, and the results will follow.

There are various online organizations where you can locate workout mates to keep you going if you need a sense of community. Also, if you live in the UK, I highly recommend Parkrun, a free walking/running event. The help has been fantastic.

Remember that losing weight is 80% diet and 20% exercise; just because you can't perform the latter doesn't imply you can't lose weight. However, physical exercise is beneficial to our entire health, so it is highly recommended that you include an exercise regimen for a healthy and sustained weight loss.

6. You believe you have failed numerous times.

So did I, and so did everyone else. Failure is frequent in many aspects of life, including attempting to lose weight. I've successfully lost and regained weight in the past for a variety of reasons.

I have yet to lose a pound in several weeks. I am honest with myself about why I failed in the first place. Maybe I didn't stick to my diet or move as much as I should have. There has to be a reason behind this; attempt to identify it and work harder this time.

It doesn't matter how many times we fail; what matters is how strong we are in rising to make it work. Get up, modify your strategy, accept your situation, be adaptable, and try again. Anything is preferable to quitting. Setting a positive mindset is extremely important, and applying it to weight loss is no exception.

7. You don't have time to enjoy yourself.

You only need to give yourself 30 minutes per day. That's nothing compared to how much time you waste looking through social media or Telegram. In fact, you can exercise at home while watching television.

Consider how much time you spend lying in bed in the mornings playing phone games. A great workout session takes less time than that. You have 30 minutes if you are determined to lose weight.

Early mornings, lunch breaks, after work, or right before bedtime are all acceptable times to exercise. If you're a busy parent with a child, consider walking while pushing the stroller for a more effective workout.

Any change in life requires some level of sacrifice, therefore if you don't have time now, it's time to sacrifice and cut back on other activities to care for your own health.

You are unmotivated.

Drops in motivation are typically one of the most difficult challenges to losing weight in many of our lives, and they are even more difficult to explain. But the good news is that if you've acknowledged a lack of motivation, you're ready to pursue solutions and fight to overcome it.

The first step is to take a break and talk to yourself if something in your life is becoming too much and is demotivating you. Perhaps taking a break can help you return stronger. But make sure the break isn't too long that it completely derails you.

The next step is to push yourself a little harder when you don't feel like working out or sticking to a good food plan. Online forums, such as Facebook groups, have always proven really beneficial in reviving my motivation.

8. You think your life is a wreck!!.

You have an injury or a breakup, you are going through a divorce, you are trying to cope as a single parent, you are fighting disease, you are facing a financial crisis, and you are mentally down all of the time. Life may be really complicated. I understand since I've been there.

To lose weight, we must accept our situation and align our goals properly. Take a break and consider what is essential to you. If you are reading this post, it is possible that losing weight is really important to you.

These hurdles to losing weight are normal for many people, yet consider how few people succeed. That is not due to a lack of failure. This is due to the fact that they conquered those challenges and prioritized their own health.

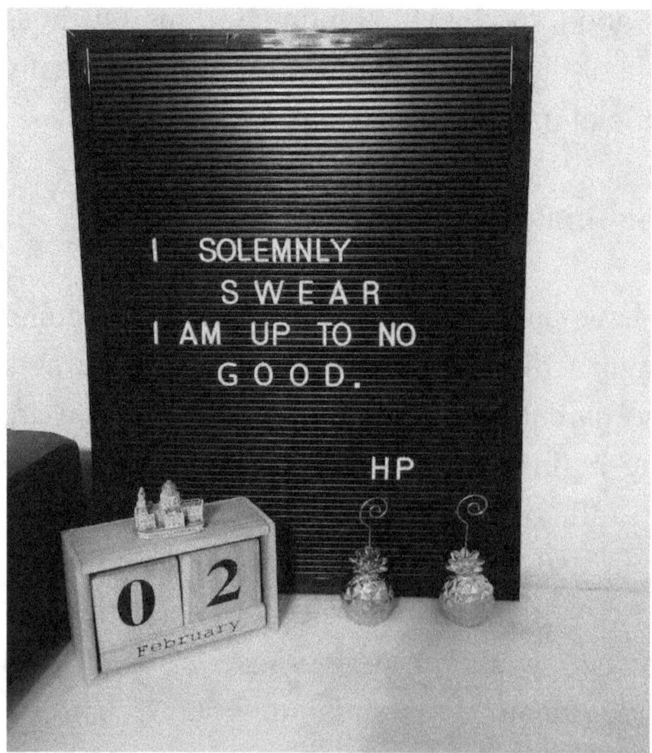

CHAPTER 7

Maintaining Your Progress

To maintain your weight, you must consume the same number of calories that you burn over the day. You should avoid making drastic changes to your diet and fitness habits. Instead, make small changes that will not result in significant weight gain. Allow yourself 6 to 8 weeks to reach your maintenance level.

Some people may discover that reducing weight is significantly easier than maintaining weight loss. Maintaining weight takes a lot of time and effort. That is why it is critical to create a plan that will assist you in maintaining your weight loss and reaching your health objectives.

Remember, too, that those who stick to a low-fat diet with plenty of fruits and vegetables are more likely to lose weight permanently. According to research, persons who are successful at sustaining their weight loss also exercise more. Here are some extra techniques to help you maintain your weight and progress to the next stage of your health journey.

Regular exercise is essential.

Whether you used exercise to help you lose weight or not, you could benefit from including regular physical activity into your day. That's because you lost weight by successfully creating a continuous calorie deficit.

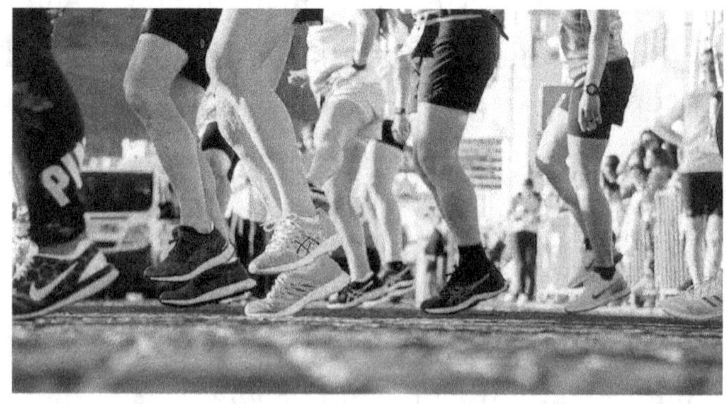

When you modify your habits, your calorie deficit may disappear and your risk of weight gain increases. Exercising frequently improves the quantity of calories you burn, which helps to prevent undesirable weight gain. This is referred to as energy balance.13

The Centers for Disease Control and Prevention (CDC) recommends that individuals engage in at least 150 minutes of moderate-intensity physical activity per week, with two days of strength training workouts.14 You may spread this out over the week as you see fit. Remember that the best workout is the one you will really do, so choose something you enjoy doing.

Watch What You Eat

People frequently revert to their old eating habits after losing weight. This is a certain method to gain weight and increases the likelihood of weight cycling. The finest meal plan is one that you can stick to for the rest of your life.

There are numerous methods to be careful of what you consume. For example, tracking your diet or calculating calories can help you monitor what you consume and support your goals.15 These steps, however, are not for everyone. In some cases, they might lead to undesirable ideas and behaviors.

If you believe that these activities may be harmful to you, you should consult with a mental health practitioner or a certified dietician. It may also be beneficial to experiment with mindful or intuitive eating habits, in which you pay attention to what you are eating and relish every bite. Furthermore, intuitive eating is based on liberating people from harmful food attitudes in order to achieve judgment-free eating.

When you practice intuitive eating, you are learning to respond to bodily hunger and satiety cues rather than emotional ones. This practice will also assist you in learning to recognize hunger, fullness, and satisfaction sensations. If you want to learn more about mindful or intuitive eating, you should speak with a mental health practitioner or registered dietitian who is skilled in these areas.

Use the 80/20 Rule.

A sustainable meal plan includes items you enjoy. It is a combination of nutritious foods that keep you full and content, with some comfort foods thrown in for good measure. The 80/20 rule states that 80% of your meals should be balanced and nutritious, while the remaining 20% should include less healthful foods.16

This may include eating balanced meals during the week and enjoying pizza night with your family on Fridays, or having a drink or two with your mates on the weekends. The objective is to acquire the perspective that all foods have a place in a well-balanced diet.

Consider Strength Training

Though many people identify strength training with muscle gain, it can also be used for weight loss and weight maintenance. That's because having more muscle means burning more calories even when you're not doing it. Strength exercise also promotes energy balance and can help avoid weight gain.

CHAPTER 8

Keeping Motivated

What inspires you to lose weight varies from person to person. still, discovering your provocation can number understanding the reasons you want to reduce weight, defining your prospects, and seeking help. Starting and sticking to a good weight loss strategy might be delicate at times. People constantly warrant drive to begin or lose provocation to continue. Fortunately, provocation can be bettered.

1. Determine Why You Want to Lose Weight.

Write down all of the reasons you ask to reduce weight. This will help you stay devoted and motivated to attain your weight loss pretensions. Try to read over them on a diurnal base and use them as a memorial when you're tempted to diverge from your weight reduction plans. Your provocations could include precluding diabetes, keeping up with grandchildren, looking your stylish for an event, enhancing your tone-confidence, or fitting into a certain brace of pants. numerous people begin losing weight because their croaker

suggests it, but exploration shows that people are more successful when their weight reduction alleviation comes from within(1Trusted Source).

2. Have Realistic prospects.

numerous diets and diet results promise quick and royal weight loss. still, utmost croakers

endorse simply slipping 1- 2 pounds(0.5- 1 kg) every week. Setting unreasonable pretensions might lead to passions of dissatisfaction and eventual failure. Setting and achieving attainable pretensions, on the other hand, produces passions of accomplishment. likewise, those who achieve their tone- determined weight loss objects are more likely to maintain their weight loss over time. A exploration that used data from multitudinous weight loss centers discovered that women who planned to lose the most weight were the most likely to drop out of the program. The good news is that indeed a small weight loss of 5- 10 of your body weight can have a significant influence on yourhealth.However, that's only 9- 18 pounds(4- 8 kg), It's 13- 25 pounds(6- 11 kg) if you weigh 250 pounds(113 kg). In fact, dwindling 5- 10 of your body weight can

• Ameliorate blood sugar control

• Reduce the threat of heart complaint

• Lower cholesterol situations

• Reduce common discomfort

• Reduce the chance of some malice

3. Concentrate on Process objects.

numerous people who are trying to lose weight simply establish outgrowth objects, or pretensions they hope to achieve at the end. generally, an outgrowth ideal will be your end target weight. still, fastening just on result pretensions can undermine your provocation. They can be too distant and leave you feeling overwhelmed. rather, identify process pretensions, or the way you will take to get your intended outgrowth. A process ideal might be to exercise four times each week. A study of 126 fat women sharing in a weight reduction program discovered that those who were process concentrated were more likely to lose weight and less likely to diverge from their diets than those who concentrated solely on weight loss pretensions. To establish solid pretensions, consider using SMART pretensions. SMART daises for

• Specific

• Measurable

• Attainable

• Realistic

• Time- bound SMART pretensions include the following exemplifications Coming week, I plan to walk for 30 twinkles five days a week. This week, I plan to consume four servings of vegetables per day. This week, I'll limit myself just one soda pop.

4. elect a plan that's applicable for your life.

Find a weight loss strategy that you can stick to and avoid bones that are virtually insolvable to follow in the long run. While there are hundreds of different diets, the maturity are centered on calorie restriction. Overeating, particularly yo- yo overeating, has been demonstrated to be a predictor of unborn weight gain. As a result, avoid rigid diets that fully remove particular foods. According to studies, people who have a" all or nothing" intelligence are less likely to lose weight. rather, try establishing your own individualized plan. The following food habits have been shown to help you lose weight. Calorie restriction Portion control Snack frequence reduction limiting fried foods and goodies Including fruits and veggies

5. Keep a Weight Loss Journal Self-monitoring.

is essential for weight loss provocation and success. People who track their food input are more likely to lose weight and keep it off, according to exploration. To keep a food journal duly, you must write down everything you consume. This includes lunches, snacks, and the chocolates you stole from your colleague's office. You can also note your feelings in your food journal. This might help you discover specific triggers for gluttony and find healthy styles to manage. You can keep a mess journal on paper or on a website or app. They've each been demonstrated to be effective

CHAPTER 9

Creating a Support System.

When making major changes in your life, it's helpful to have the support of those around you. Because long- term weight loss success will include adaptations in your eating habits and life, numerous people find that having the support of medical professionals, family members, and musketeers may be a significant tool as they try to reduce weight. Medical weight loss can give a significant quantum of support while you fight to achieve your pretensions, but it can also be salutary to meat out your support system with people in your regular life. To begin constructing a support structure that will make long- term weight loss simpler, Your Weight Loss Center Checking in with a croaker

and medical platoon on a regular base can give redundant incitement and the direction demanded to maintain weight loss for numerous people. We will be then to help you from the moment you start one of our weight loss programs. still, please communicate us via our website or call one of our services so we can help you in chancing a result, If you have any enterprises or problems. musketeers and family musketeers and family members can help you keep motivated and responsible because they're the people you'll interact with every day. By informing these folks about the advancements you want to make, you will have a whole platoon of people lodging for you to succeed. Begin by telling these people how they can help you. Ask them to join you for healthy refections or to be your drill mate. You might also request that they cease doing conditioning that make it delicate for you to lose weight, similar as incinerating eyefuls every week. The people you live with will be the most vital to bandy your new life with. Ask everybody who lives with you to be probative and positive about your bournes . Make a rule to keep junk food out of the house. Your actions may rub off on these folks, inspiring them to join you in your healthy conditioning. The World Wide Web The Internet is an excellent source of information and help for nearly any problem you may be facing. Using forums and social media groups can give you with a global support system, allowing you to seek advice and help from other people who are trying to reduce weight and may have gone through analogous gests as you. Our Facebook runner is a atrocious position to meet other people going through medical weight loss in Los Angeles and Bakersfield. You can also look for other weight loss- related groups on Facebook or produce your own. It can also help to probe or ask questions on websites with forums, similar asmyfitnesspal.com. It'll be simpler to stay motivated and make the life changes needed to lose weight and keep it off if you have a strong support system behind you.

CHAPTER 10

Embracing a Healthy and Happy You.

Losing weight can be a difficult task, both physically and mentally. While it is critical to prioritize your health and well-being, it is also critical to practice self-love and acceptance throughout the process. After all, a good body image may be a powerful motivator and can help you maintain your weight loss objectives in the long run. Here's how to accept yourself as you are while on a weight-loss journey:

Fall in Love With Your Body:

Instead of focusing on what you don't like about your physique, concentrate on what you do. Remember that your body is magnificent and deserves to be acknowledged.

Take time each day to show thanks to your body.

Find something to be grateful for, whether it's your strong legs that get you through your workouts or your healthy heart that keeps you going.

When you're dealing with self-doubt or negative self-talk, treat yourself with care and compassion. Speak to yourself as you would to a loved one, and remember that you are deserving of love and respect.

Surround Yourself with Positivity: Surround yourself with people, images, and messages that elevate and encourage you. This might be following body-positive social media accounts, joining a supportive community, or spending time with friends that encourage you.

Set attainable objectives:

Setting realistic goals is essential for keeping motivation and building confidence. Instead of focusing on a certain number on the scale, make incremental, long-term improvements that will enhance your overall health.

Celebrate Your Progress:

Celebrate your progress, no matter how tiny. Whether it's fitting into a pair of trousers that previously didn't fit or running an extra mile, take time to recognize and appreciate your accomplishments.

Self-care is an act of self-love. Make time for leisure and relaxation, prioritize good habits like getting adequate sleep and staying hydrated, and engage in things that make you joyful.

Remember that accepting yourself as you are does not imply complacency. It entails admitting and accepting where you are while striving for a healthier, happier you.

Conclusion

"Slimming Strategies: Unlocking the Secrets to a Healthier, Happier You" contains a plethora of efficient strategies and time-tested approaches to reducing unwanted pounds and attaining long-term effects. From significant mindset shifts to tailored nutrition programs and energizing exercise routines, this comprehensive book provides you with the skills and knowledge you need to embark on a successful journey toward your optimum weight and better well-being. Discover the transformation that awaits you as you unleash the potential within and embrace a new chapter in your life full with confidence, vigor, and self-love.